# RESTORE YOUR
## HEALTH
### BY JUICING NATURAL VEGETABLES AND FRUITS

JOSEPH  THOMPSON

ISBN:1725094533
ISBN-13: 9781725094536

# DEDICATION

This book is dedicated to my grandmother Sarah Thompson and my Grandfather Vincent Haynes. I love you both and I want to thank you even though you are not here on Earth I know you are watching over me. Grandpa thank you for building me my first cabinet so I could hang up my clothes I will never let you down and I promise to make you proud one day.

THIS PAGE WAS LEFT BLANK INTENTIONALLY

# THE FUNDAMENTALS OF HOME JUICING

Restoring your health is the best thing you can do for your mind and body. I remember my grandmother making natural carrot juice for me and my dad at dinner and it was so good. I use to watch both her and my mother use a blender to make these juices and I thought to myself boy I wish I could that now that I am older I juice my carrots just like my grandmother did and I reap all the rewards from living this healthy lifestyle. One of my favorite is carrot and orange with apples it's so smooth and easy to go down some of the recipes are in this book.  It's quiet easy to do with any standard blender or juicer, you can juice almost any fruit or vegetable into a tasty drink. Not only will you extract more juice from apples, lemons, oranges. You will get more nutrients and healthier stuff if you juice them. Those who like juices believe that the lack of fiber permits nutrients to be absorbed easier and faster into the body. In order to make your own juices all you need is just a blender and a strainer or small juicer. The recipes in this book require a either one of these two kitchen appliances the price for one of these are fairly moderate ranges from 15-29 dollars.

## IMPORTANT THINGS TO DO BEFORE YOU JUICE

Always wash your vegetables and fruits before you begin to juice you always want to make sure your fruits are clean there are many bacteria that can be harboring on your apple so peeling it might not be such a bad idea. Carrots can be scraped and then cut up into small pieces and then placed in the blender. You can also use vinegar to wash your fruits and vegetables cold water or hot water can also kill bacteria harboring on the leaves and skin of your fresh produce. E.coli  and other harmful pesticides will be removed if you take the time to properly clean and prepare your produce before juicing them.

## SMOOTHIES VS JUICE

Smoothies are usually fruits blend with yogurt ice or almond milk or soy. Juices however are just raw fruits and vegetables blended up with water or any extra additives you decide to add; both provide great health benefits. You can experiment with all kinds of fruits even nuts and berries to get the taste you are looking for some are sour and some are sweet so make the best choice.

## FRUITS THAT PROVIDE GREAT HEALTH BENEFITS
1. Mango
2. Apples
3. Oranges
4. Watermelon
5. Kiwi
6. Tangerine
7. Grapefruit
8. Strawberries
9. Grapes
10. Cantaloupes
11. Pineapples
12. Aloe
13. Coconuts
14. Peach
15. Pears

## VEGETABLES THAT PROVIDE GREAT HEALTH BENEFITS

1. Kale
2. Cabbage
3. Carrots
4. Wheat Grass
5. Broccoli
6. Celery
7. Bok Choy
8. Cucumber
9. Corn
10. Spinach
11. Lettice

THIS PAGE WAS LEFT BLANK INTENTIONALLY

# CONTENTS


|  | Acknowledgments | i |
|---|---|---|
| 1 | HEALTHIER HEART & LIVER............... | 3 |
| 2 | BETTER VISION.................................. | Pg 4 |
| 3 | FATIGUE............................................. | Pg 5 |
| 4 | NASAL PROBLEMS............................... | Pg 6 |
| 5 | STRONGER BONES............................... | Pg 7 |
| 6 | FIGHT THE CANCER............................. | Pg 8 |
| 7 | FIXING MIGRAINES............................. | Pg 9 |
| 8 | JUICES FOR BREATHING PROBLEMS..... | Pg 10 |
| 9 | STOMACH PROBLEMS.......................... | Pg 11 |
| 10 | DEALING WITH HIGH BLOOD PRESSURE | Pg 12 |
| 11 | HIGH CHOLESTEROL........................... | Pg 13 |
| 12 | HYPERTENSION................................. | Pg 14 |
| 13 | HEALTHIER SMILE.............................. | Pg 15 |
| 14 | CALCIUM.......................................... | Pg 16 |
| 15 | IRON................................................. | Pg 17 |
| 16 | ZINC................................................. | Pg 18 |
| 17 | MAGNESIUM...................................... | Pg 19 |
| 18 | POTASSIUM....................................... | Pg 20 |
| 19 | PHOSPHORUS.................................... | Pg 21 |
| 20 | COPPER............................................. | Pg 22 |

Joseph Thompson

x

THIS PAGE WAS LEFT BLANK INTENTIONALLY

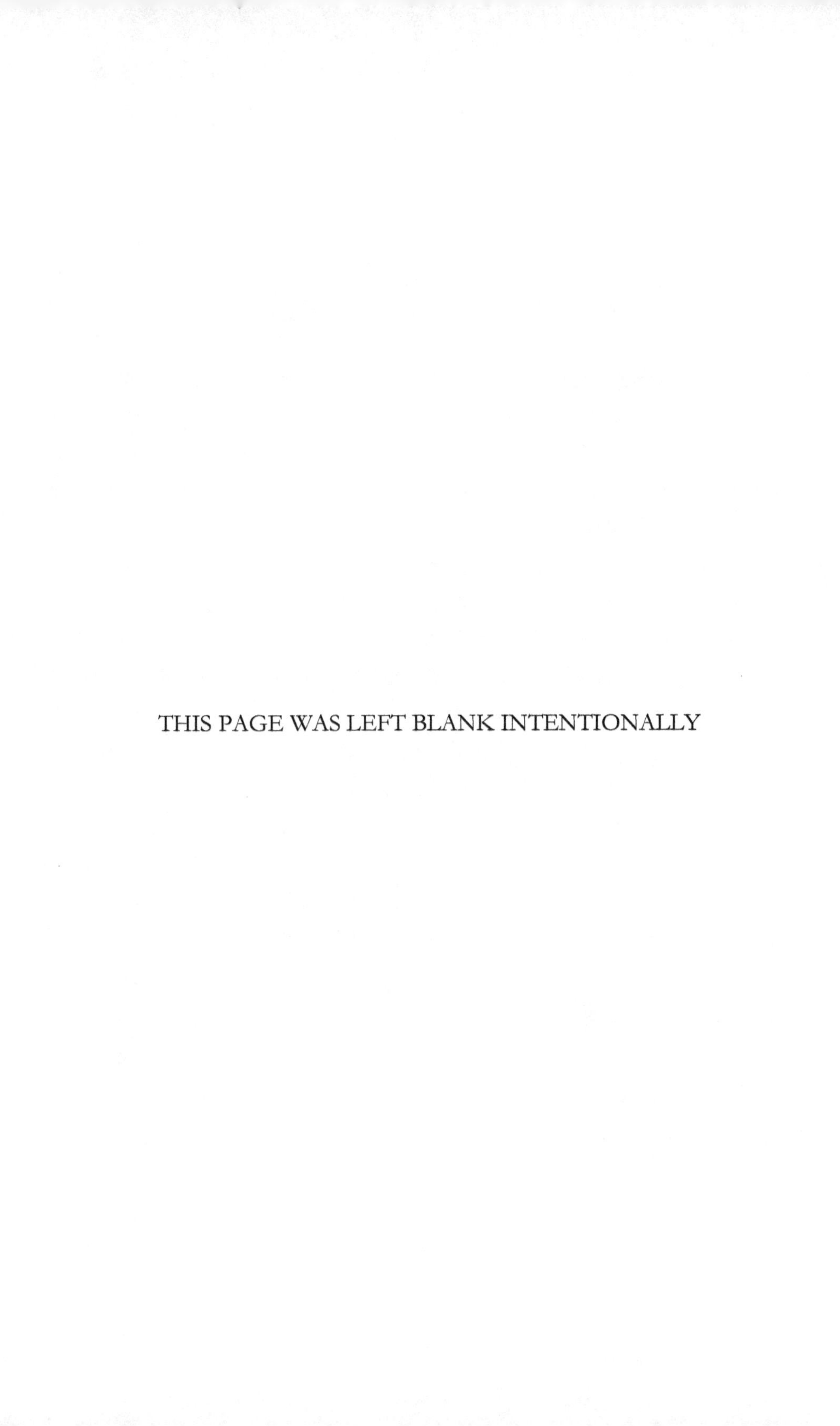

THIS PAGE WAS LEFT BLANK INTENTIONALLY

# ACKNOWLEDGMENTS

Thanks to my mother for teaching me how to live right and eat healthy. I will be forever in your debt.

Joseph Thompson

ii

THIS PAGE WAS LEFT BLANK INTENTIONALLY

# HEALTHIER HEART & LIVER

## HEART DISEASE
Carrot
Beet
Broccoli

---

## LIVER PROBLEMS
Carrot
Apple
Beets

---

# 2
# BETTER VISION
4

## EYES & VISION PROBLEMS
Carrot
Celery

---

## NIGHT BLINDNESS
Carrot
Apple

# FATIGUE
Carrot
Spinach

---

# NERVOUSNESS
Carrot
Celery

# 4
# NASAL PROBLEMS

## COLDS
Carrot
Ginger
Beet
Cucumber

---

## SORE THROAT
Carrot
Apple
Parsley
Ginger

---

## ALLERGY SUFFERS
Carrot
Beets
Spinach
Celery

---

## SINUS PROBLEMS
Carrot
Papaya

# 5
# STRONGER BONES

## BONE BUILDING TONIC

Carrot
Apple
Parsley
Kale

---

## ANEMIA

Carrot
Beets
Spinach
Kalé

---

## MUSCLE CRAMPS

Carnot
Spinach
Parsley

6
FIGHT THE CANCER

# CANCER
Carrot
Broccoli
Apple
Wheat Grass

# 7
# FIXING MIGRAINES

# HEADACHES
Carrot
Beet
Cucumbers

# 8
# JUICES FOR BREATHING PROBLEMS

## ASTHMA
Carrot
Celery

# STOMACH PROBLEMS

## ACID STOMACH

Carrot
Beets
Cucumber

---

## UPSET STOMACH

Carrot
Apple
Parsley

---

## ULCERS

Carrot
Cabbage
Celery

---

## GOUT

Carrot
Celery
Parsley

---

## DIGESTION PROBLEM

Carrot
Apples

---

## IRREGULARITY

Carrot
Apple
Celery
Wheat Grass

# 10
# DEALING WITH HIGH BLOOD PRESSURE

## HIGH BLOOD PRESSURE
Carrot
Parsley
Celery
Garlic

---

## LOW BLOOD PRESSURE
Carrot
Spinach
Celery

# 11
# HIGH CHOLESTEROL

# HIGH CHOLESTEROL
Carrot
Apple
Parsley

12
HYPERTENSION

# HYPERTENSION
Carrot
Beets
Spinach

---

# IMPOTENCY
Carrot
Broccoli
Cabbage
Kale

# 13
# HEALTHIER SMILE

## TOOTH DECAY
Carrot
Parsley
Kale

# 14
# CALCIUM

# CALCIUM
Carrot
Broccoli
Kale
Parsley

# 15
# IRON

# IRON
Carrot
Apple
Spinach

16
ZINC

# ZINC
Carrot
Apple
Parsley
Ginger

17
MAGNESIUM

# MAGNESIUM

Carrot
Apple
Beets
Broccoli

18
POTASSIUM

# POTASSIUM
Strawberry

# 19 PHOSPHORUS

## PHOSPHORUS
Carrots
Cauliflower
Parsley
Grape
Tangerine

# 20 COOPER

# COOPER
Carrots
Potato
Swiss Chard

---

# SODIUM
Carrots
Celery
Spinach

---

# SILICON
Carrots
Celery
Grape
Parsley
Apples

---

# SULFUR
Carrots
Apple
Cabbage
Kalé

# ABOUT THE AUTHOR

Joseph Thompson
Graduate of Lincoln University
Sports enthusiast, Practice healthy living